Table of Contents

Lymphoma is cancer that begins in infection-fighting cells of the immune system, called lymphocytes. These cells are in the lymph nodes, spleen, thymus, bone marrow, and other parts of the body. When you have lymphoma, lymphocytes change and grow out of control.

There are two main types of lymphoma:

Non-Hodgkin: Most people with lymphoma have this type.

Hodgkin

Non-Hodgkin and Hodgkin lymphoma involve different types of lymphocyte cells. Every type of lymphoma grows at a different rate and responds differently to treatment.

Lymphoma is very treatable, and the outlook can vary depending on the type of lymphoma and its stage. Your doctor can help you find the right treatment for your type and stage of the illness.

Lymphoma is different from leukemia. Each of these cancers starts in a different type of cell.

Lymphoma starts in infection-fighting lymphocytes.

Leukemia starts in blood-forming cells inside bone marrow.

BREAKFAST

1. Rustic Eggplant Moussaka

Prep Time: 60 Minutes

Cook Time: 120 Minutes

Servings: 8

Ingredients

- 3 lbs Eggplant (2 extra-large or 3 eggplants)
- Salt
- 3 tablespoons olive oil or cooking spray
- Tomato Meat Sauce:
- 2 tablespoons olive oil
- 1 large onion, diced
- 4 cloves garlic, rough chopped
- 2 lbs ground lamb, ground beef (or use vegetarian ground meat substitute -Gimme Lean or St Ives Meatless Ground.) I prefer lamb.
- 1 ½ cups diced tomatoes, with juices (or 14-ounce can, with juices)

- 3 tablespoons tomato paste
- ½ cup white wine (optional, sub 1/4 cup water)
- 2 teaspoons dried oregano
- 1 tsp sugar
- 1 tsp cinnamon
- 3/4 tsp kosher salt
- 1/2 teaspoon cracked pepper
- 2–3 tablespoons fresh chopped parsley

Bechamel Sauce:

- 3 tablespoons butter or olive oil
- 4 tablespoons flour
- 2 cups milk
- 1/2 tsp nutmeg (use fresh grated if possible)
- 1/4 tsp kosher salt
- 1/8 tsp pepper or white pepper
- 1/4 cup grated Parmesan, Pecorino or Kefalotiri Cheese (plus an additional 1/4 cup for the top-optional)
- 1 egg, room temp, lightly beaten

Instructions

1. Pre-heat oven to 400 F. Cut eggplant into ⅓- ¼ inch thick disks (no thinner), sprinkle with a little kosher

salt and let sit in a colander or bowl for 20-60 minutes. Eggplant will start to release liquid (making it less bitter)

2. Rinse well, pat dry and brush each side with olive oil (or use spray oil).

3. Place on a greased sheet pan and roast in a 400 F oven until golden, about 20-30 minutes. Alternatively, you can grill the eggplant on each side (getting nice deep grill marks) then wrapping it in foil after for 10-15 minutes, so it steams and cooks through.

4. While eggplant is roasting -make the tomato- meat sauce: In a large pan, saute diced onion in oil on med-high heat for 3-4 minutes, add garlic, turn heat down to med-low and saute for 8-10 minutes until onions are tender. Add the ground lamb (or beef or vegetarian meat), turn heat up to medium and brown, stirring often, about 15 minutes. Drain fat if any. Add the rest of the ingredients -diced tomatoes, tomato paste, white wine, fresh chopped parsley, sugar, cinnamon, kosher salt and pepper. Stir and cover and let simmer on med-low heat for 20 minutes.

5. Make Bechamel Sauce: In a small pot, heat the butter. Whisk in the flour and let cook for 2-3 minutes on med heat, stirring often. Whisk in the first cup of milk a little

at a time. Whisk well, and add the 2nd cup. Stirring constantly bring to a boil, lower heat, and let simmer on low for an additional 2 minutes. Remove from heat and add nutmeg, cheese, salt, pepper. Set aside to cool. In a separate bowl, lightly beat an egg, but do not add it just yet.

6. Assemble: Divide eggplant slices into three stacks, reserving the best looking largest pieces for the top and bottom layers. The others can be placed in the middle layer which will be concealed.

7. In a greased 8x 13 inch baking dish, place one layer of eggplant. Add half the meat sauce. Add another layer of eggplant and the remaining meat sauce. Add the third and final layer of eggplant. Whisk in 2-3 tablespoons of bechamel sauce, into the beaten egg (to temper it) then pour this into the bechamel sauce, whisking until nice and smooth. Spread the bechamel over the final eggplant layer.

8. Sprinkle with the remaining cheese (optional) and place in a 350F oven for 50-60 minutes, uncovered until beautifully golden. Let stand 10 minutes before serving.

Prep Time: 15 Minutes

Cook Time: 60 Minutes

Servings: 6

Ingredients

- 3 Japanese eggplant or one large eggplant
- 1 red or yellow bell pepper
- 2 medium tomatoes
- 2 zucchini or summer squash
- 1 onion
- 8–14 garlic cloves, whole, peeled
- 2–3 tablespoon fresh herbs – thyme or rosemary or combination of both
- Olive oil for drizzling
- Salt and pepper to taste
- Splash balsamic vinegar
- Optional Garnishes: Italian parsley or fresh basil ribbons, capers, chili flakes, olive oil
- Serve with pasta, soft polenta, whole grains, or feel free to add beans, sausage, and chicken.
- Easy Creamy Polenta

- 1 cup corn meal
- 4 ½ cups water or stock
- 1 tablespoon olive oil or butter
- ½ cup grated cheese (cheddar, Parmesan, mozzarella, goat cheese)
- Salt and pepper to taste

Instructions

1. Preheat oven to 400 F and place a piece of parchment on 1-2 large sheet pans (I use two).
2. Using a vegetable peeler, peel eggplant if you want – or just remove some of the skin in long strips. Or if you prefer, leave the skin on. Cut into ½ inch thick bite-sized pieces. Slice the bell pepper into ½ inch wide strips. Cut the tomatoes into 3/4 inch wedges. Slice the zucchini the long way and then slice into ½ inch thick half-moons. Slice the onion into ¼-½ inch thick half-moons.
3. Spread out the veggies on the sheet pan in a single layer (this is why you most likely need two sheet pans). Add whole garlic cloves (peeled) and herbs.

4. Drizzle with olive oil and toss, using enough oil to coat. Sprinkle with a generous amount of salt and pepper. Toss well.

5. Roast in the hot oven for 20 minutes, mix the veggies, roast 20 more minutes, mix again. Turn heat down to 300 and roast 10-20 more minutes, or until tender and edges begin to caramelize.

6. Taste, adjust salt, and drizzle with a little splash of balsamic vinegar.

7. Use immediately or cool and refrigerate (or freeze) until ready to use.

Prep Time: 50 Minutes

Cook Time: 45 Minutes

Servings: 6

Ingredients

- 3–4 medium eggplant (3 inches wide by 5 inches long)
- 1 lb ground lamb, ground beef, or ground plant-based "meat"
- 1 onion
- 4 garlic
- 1 1/2 teaspoons salt
- 1 teaspoon cumin
- 3/4 teaspoons allspice
- 1/2 teaspoon ground coriander
- 1/2 teaspoon sumac
- 1/2 teaspoon cinnamon
- 1/4 teaspoon ground cloves
- 1/4 teaspoon ground cardamon
- 1/4 teaspoon ground nutmeg
- 2 medium tomatoes, diced (1 1/2 cups) plus their juices
- 2 cups cooked basmati rice

- 1/4 cup fresh dill
- 1/4 cup fresh mint
- 1/4 cup pinenuts, toasted (save 1 tablespoon for garnish)
- —2 tablespoons tomato paste
- 2 cups broth- chicken, veggie, or use water and pinch salt
- 1/4 teaspoon allspice
- 1/4 teaspoon cumin
- Garnish: fresh dill and mint

Instructions

1. Prep the Eggplant: Scoop out the eggplant leaving about ½ inch thickness on all sides. I find the easiest way to do this is to use a knife around the edge, then crosshatch, and use a spoon to remove. It need not be perfect.
2. Season the eggpant shells with salt and pepper and set aside, and chop up the filling finely.
3. Preheat the oven to 400F
4. Make the filling: In a large oven-proof braiser or pan, saute the ground meat and onions over medium heat for 4-5 minutes, until onions are fragrant, then add the

diced eggplant and garlic, cooking until eggplant is translucent. Drain some fat if you like. Season with salt and all the spices. Add the fresh tomatoes and their juices, stir and cover for a few minutes until the tomatoes break down into the meat.

5. Place the meat mixture in bowl with the cooked rice, fresh herbs and optional peanuts (remembering to save a tablespoon for garnish after baking). Give a stir and adjust salt and spices to taste. (If using lentils, I would add a good drizzle of olive oil.)

6. Make the tomato broth: In the same pan, heat up the broth, tomato paste and spices and whisk, scraping up any brown bits. Wipe off the sides of the pan if messy with a wet paper towel. Turn off heat.

7. Fill the eggplant: Divide the filling among the eggplants, pressing it in gently, and mounding to incorporate all. Nestle them in the tomato broth. You can also bake these in a baking dish if you prefer. The broth should come up about ¼ – ½ inch -add more broth if necessary.

8. Bake the Eggplant: 400F –covered, 40-45 minutes, until eggplant is fork tender, and filling is heated through (145F), then bake uncovered for 5-10 minutes, until golden.

9. Garnish: Sprinkle with fresh dill and mint and remaining peanuts. TIP: Whenever I serve peanuts to people who I don't know well or am not sure of allergies- I always make them visible, on top.

Prep Time: 30 Minutes

Cook Time: 40 Minutes

Servings: 6

Ingredients

- 1 extra-large eggplant (or two small)
- 2 teaspoons salt
- Bowl of water
- 2–4 tablespoons olive oil (divided) or coconut oil.
- 1 medium onion, diced
- 6–8 garlic cloves, rough chopped
- 1 cup celery
- 1 red bell pepper (or large carrot)
- 1 tablespoon, ras el hanout, more taste
- 1 teaspoon cumin
- 1 teaspoon coriander
- 1/4 teaspoon cinnamon
- 14-ounce can diced or crushed tomatoes
- 1/3 cup raisins (or chopped dried apricots)
- 1 teaspoon salt, more to taste
- 1/2 teaspoon pepper

- 14-ounce can chickpeas, drained, rinsed.
- 1 cup veggie broth
- Garnishes: Cinnamon scented couscous, flat-leaf parsley, olive oil, optional yogurt, and optional Aleppo chili flakes
- Cinnamon-Scented Couscous (serves 4)
- 1 3/4 cup veggie stock
- 1–2 tablespoons olive oil
- 1 small cinnamon stick (or 1/2 teaspoon)
- 1/2 teaspoon cumin
- 1/2 teaspoon granulated garlic (or onion)
- 1/2 teaspoon salt, more to taste
- 1 1/2 cup dry couscous

Instructions

1. Prep Eggplant: Quarter the eggplant, and cut into large chunks (1 1/2 inches at widest part). Place in a big bowl, cover with cool water just to enough to cover, and stir in the salt. Place a plate over top to keep the eggplant submerged 20 minutes. Drain and pat dry. (Don't rinse.)
2. Preheat the oven to 375F

3. Pan Sear: In a large Dutch oven, or ovenproof skillet, over medium-high heat, heat 2 tablespoons oil. Working in 2 batches, brown two sides of the eggplant, until golden, then set these aside. No need to cook through.

4. Make the stew: Add more oil to the same pan, and the onion and saute 2-3 minutes, stirring. Add the garlic, celery and red pepper and lower heat, cook until tender about 5 minutes. Lower heat to low. Add the spices, canned tomatoes (and juices), raisins, salt, pepper, chickpeas and veggie broth. Bring to simmer, stirring.

5. Nestle in the eggplant and give the pan a good shake so the stew levels. It should be like a stew-like. If it seems dry, add a little water. Drizzle with a little olive oil, cover tightly and place in the warm oven.

6. Bake 20-25 minutes or until eggplant is tender and cooked through. While it's baking make the couscous.

7. Remove the lid, taste adding more salt to taste, keeping in mind the couscous will soak up some of the salt. If you feel the stew needs more flavor overall, add a little more ras el hanout, a 1/2 teaspoon at a time, tasting as you go. If it seems watery, bake uncovered for a few minutes. If dry, add a little water. To serve, Sprinkle with optional Aleppo chili flakes and fresh Parsley. I

like adding an additional drizzle of olive oil, or a dollop of yogurt, up to you.

8. Serve with the cinnamon-scented couscous.

9. To make couscous: Place broth, oil, spices and salt in a medium pot, and bring to boil. Stir in couscous. Cover and remove from heat. Let stand 7 minutes. Uncover and fluff with fork. Adjust salt.

Prep Time: 15 Minutes

Cook Time: 90 Minutes

Servings: 8

Ingredients

- 2 pounds eggplant- Japanese, Chinese or fairytale
- 10 garlic cloves
- 2 fat shallots, quartered
- 3/4 cup olive oil
- 1 1/2 teaspoons salt
- 2 teaspoons ras el hanout or Villa Jerada Ras El Hanout
- 1 teaspoon caraway seeds (or sub fennel seeds)
- 1/2 teaspoon pepper
- 4 medium tomatoes (or 1 lb cherry tomatoes), quartered
- Large lemon zest pieces, from one lemon (use a veggie peeler or sharp knife)
- Garnish: kalamata or Moroccan olives, Italian parsley, chili flakes (like Aleppo or Urfa)

Instructions

1. Preheat oven to 375F

2. Cut eggplant in half lengthwise (or slices no thicker than 3/4 inch) and place in an ovenproof baking dish along with the whole garlic cloves and shallots.

3. In a small bowl, mix the olive oil, salt, pepper, ras el hanout, and caraway seeds.

4. Pour over the eggplant and toss well to coat. Cover with foil and bake 20 mins on the middle rack.

5. After the first 20 minutes, lower heat to 350F and uncover.

6. Add the tomatoes, zest and give a toss.

7. Continue baking 50-75 minutes, uncovered, checking every 20 minutes, giving a gentle stir, until the eggplant is meltingly tender and creamy. Depending on the eggplant size, the time may vary. Please be patient here and check more often if eggplants are very small.

8. Once the eggplant is very tender, and the edges are crisp, pull it out of the oven, cover lightly with foil until ready to serve. Garnish with the olives, fresh herbs and optional chili flakes. Serve warm or at room temp.

Prep Time: 15 Minutes

Cook Time: 45 Minutes

Servings: 3

Ingredients

- 3 lb Spaghetti Squash- (or sub pasta noodles)
- 4 tablespoons olive oil– divided
- 1 medium eggplant – cut into a small dice (4 cups)
- 1 red onion- diced
- 4–6 cloves garlic- rough chopped
- 1 red bell pepper- diced
- 14 ounce can crushed or diced tomatoes
- 1 tablespoon dry Italian herbs (or sub oregano and thyme)
- 1 teaspoon kosher salt
- ¼ teaspoon red chili flakes, more to taste
- Splash red wine
- 2 tablespoons capers, more to taste, plus a splash of the brine
- 3 tablespoons slice olives (like green or kalamata)

- Garnish: fresh Italian parsley, grated Romano or Parmesan cheese, or a drizzle olive oil

Instructions

1. Preheat oven to 425F

2. Cut squash in half widthwise, place open side down, on a parchment-lined baking sheet in the oven and roast for 30- 40 minutes (depending on size) or until knife tender. Turn on their sides, allowing steam to escape, continue roasting 5-10 minutes, so they dry out a bit.

3. While the squash is roasting make the Eggplant Puttanesca sauce.

4. In a large heavy bottom skillet or dutch oven, heat 3 tablespoons oil over med-high heat. Add diced onion and eggplant, and saute, stirring often for 4-5 minutes. Add garlic and red bell pepper, turn heat down to medium and continue cooking until eggplant is tender, about 10-12 more minutes, stirring occasionally.

5. Add crushed tomatoes, a generous splash of wine, chili flakes, salt, pepper, Italian herbs, and simmer on low heat 5-10 more minutes. Add capers and olives.

6. Taste, adjust salt, spice level and add more capers or olives to taste. Sometimes I'll add a little splash of the caper or olive brine, to bump up the flavor.

7. When spaghetti squash is tender, scoop the seeds out- then scoop out spaghetti squash strands into a bowl, and fluff and toss well with salt, pepper and 1 tablespoon olive oil.

8. Divide among bowls and top with the eggplant puttanesca. Sprinkle with fresh Italian parsley and grated cheese (optional) or drizzle olive oil.

9. Alternatively, you can serve this right out of the spaghetti squash shell (making sure to season the squash, mixing with a fork before topping with the putttanesca.

Prep Time: 25 Minutes

Cook Time: 45 Minutes

Servings: 6

Ingredients

- 1 ½ cups cooked quinoa (or sub rice, cauliflower "rice", cous cous, orzo or other grain)
- 3 large red bell peppers
- ½ an onion
- 1 tablespoon olive oil
- 2 small Japanese eggplant, diced (or sub zucchini) about 2 cups
- 4 garlic cloves, rough chopped
- 1 can chickpeas, drained (or sub 1 1/2 cups salted, browned, ground beef, turkey, lamb or chicken)
- 1–2 tablespoon za'atar spice (or sub 11/2 teaspoon cumin, 1 1/2 tsp coriander, 1 1/2 tsp sesame seeds)
- Salt and pepper to taste.
- Zest of one small lemon
- ½ cup chopped Italian parsley, more for garnish (or cilantro)

- Garnish: Zhoug Yogurt –my favorite! (See notes), pine nuts or slivered almonds

Instructions

1. Set the quinoa to cook. Preheat the oven to 400F.
2. Preheat the grill to high heat to grill the peppers. (Alternatively, you can roast these- see notes).
3. Cut peppers in half lengthwise and grill them on each side for about 6-7 minutes or until tender, and a little charred. (They will soften more in the oven later)
4. While peppers are grilling, heat oil in a large skillet and sauté the onion and eggplant over medium heat until eggplant is tender. Add the garlic and another little drizzle of oil if needed and cook 2 more minutes until garlic is fragrant. Add the chickpeas (or cooked meat) and quinoa and season generously with the zaatar spice. Taste, and add more to taste.
5. Season generously with salt and pepper. Add lemon zest and parsley. Taste and adjust salt and seasonings. If the mixture seems dry add a splash of water to loosen just slightly.
6. Place peppers in a baking dish and divide the filling among them, packing and mounding them up high.

Cover with foil and bake for 25 minutes, remove foil, and bake for 10 more minutes.

7. Spoon the flavorful Zhoug yogurt over top, or serve on the side. Garnish with more parsley and optional pine nuts.

Prep Time: 15 Minutes

Cook Time: 60 Minutes

Servings: 2

Ingredients

- 1 globe eggplant (about 1– 1 ⅛ lb)
- 1 ½ tablespoons olive oil
- 1 tablespoon zataar spice mix- or see notes (or use store-bought zaatar!)
- ¼ teaspoon salt, more to taste
- 1 fat garlic clove
- Served with:
- 2 cups cooked rice or grains (freekeh, farro, and quinoa)
- 1–2 cups fresh chopped veggies- tomato, cucumber, radish, grated carrot or beets
- Your choice of tahini sauce, plain yogurt, or tzatziki
- Other options- Italian parsley, kalamata olives, Aleppo chili flakes, feta or goat cheese crumbles

Instructions

1. Preheat oven to 400F

2. Slice Eggplant in half, then slice deeply at a diagonal at
    one-inch intervals -"crosshatching" (see photos above)
    careful not to cut through skin.

3. Season each side with ⅛ teaspoon kosher salt,
    sprinkling it into the slices if possible.

4. Mix oil, spices, garlic together in a bowl to make a
    paste. Brush or spoon the entire contents over the
    eggplant and place on a sheet pan in the oven and bake
    for 1 hour rotating halfway through. After an hour,
    pierce with a fork and if they are very tender and juicy,
    they are done. Bigger eggplants may take longer.

5. In the meantime, cook the grain and chop or prep any
    other veggies.

6. When the eggplant is done, assemble the plates,
    topping the warm rice or grain with the roasted
    eggplant, then surround with fresh veggies and drizzle
    with tahini sauce, yogurt or tzatziki– or you could
    simply season the fresh veggies and rice with salt,
    lemon and olive oil. Add olives or cheese if you wish.
    Sprinkle with fresh Italian parsley. Enjoy!

Prep Time: 20 Minutes

Cook Time: 25 Minutes

Servings: 4

Ingredients

- 1 1/2 lbs Japanese Eggplant (about 4 x 10 inch eggplants)
- 2 teaspoons salt
- Bowl of water
- —-2 tablespoons cornstarch
- 2–4 tablespoons peanut oil (or wok oil)
- —4 cloves garlic, rough chopped
- 2 teaspoons ginger, finely minced
- 5–10 dried red chilies

Szechuan Sauce:

- 1 teaspoon Szechuan peppercorns (or sub regular peppercorns)
- 1/4 cup soy sauce or low sodium soy sauce
- 1 tablespoon garlic chili paste (or sub 1 teaspoon chili flakes)

- 1 tablespoon sesame oil

- 1 tablespoon rice vinegar

- 1 tablespoon Chinese cooking wine (or mirin)

- 3 tablespoons sugar, brown sugar, coconut sugar, maple syrup or alternative

- 1/2 teaspoon five spice

- Garnish with scallions and roasted peanuts or this Peanut Chili crunch

Instructions

1. Cut eggplant into 1/2 inch thick half-moons or into bite-sized pieces (see photos). Place in a big bowl covered with water and stir in 2 teaspoons salt. Cover with a plate and let stand 20-30 minutes.

2. In the meantime, chop the garlic and ginger and make the Szechuan Sauce.

3. To make the Szechuan Sauce: Toast the Szechuan peppercorns in a dry skillet over medium heat for 1-2 minutes. Crush. Place these along with the remaining ingredients (soy, chili paste, sesame oil, rice vinegar, Chinese cooking wine, sugar, and five spice) in a small bowl and whisk. Set by the stove.

4. Drain and rinse the eggplant and pat dry with a towel. Toss with the corn starch.

5. Working in 2 batches, heat 1 -2 tablespoons oil in an extra-large skillet over medium heat. Add half the eggplant spreading them out. You want to get both sides nice and golden, and the insides cooked through -so take your time here and don't rush this step. Let one side brown then turn them over using tongs. This will take about 10 minutes for each batch. (If in a hurry sometimes I'll use 2 pans.) Set the eggplant aside.

6. Add 1 more tablespoon oil to the skillet, and over medium heat, add the garlic and ginger, stirring for 2 minutes. Turn the fan on, add the dried chills and stir one minute. Pour the Szechuan sauce into the pan and bring to a simmer for 20 seconds. Add the eggplant back into the skillet, tossing gently for about 1 minute. If it seems dry add a tablespoon of water to loosen.

7. Place in a serving dish and top with scallions and optional peanuts.

8. Serve with rice, cauliflower rice, black rice or rice noodles.

Prep Time: 15 Minutes

Cook Time: 30 Minutes

Servings: 4

Ingredients

- 1 pound eggplants, sliced long and thin. Use 2 Chinese or Japanese eggplants or 1 large Globe eggplant.
- 3– 4 tablespoons coconut oil (or peanut, or other high heat oil)
- 1 1/2 tablespoons garlic, roughly chopped
- 1–6 fresh Thai chilis, finely diced (optional, or sub milder chilies like jalapeno, or red chili paste)
- 1 pound chicken, thinly sliced. Use any protein of choice (crispy tofu, ground turkey, shrimp, etc.)
- 1/2 cup onion, sliced
- 1/2 cup bell peppers, bite-sized pieces
- 1/2 cup pea pods, chopped into 2-3 inch pieces (or sub more bell pepper)
- 1 cup Thai Basil (or sub regular basil)
- 1 tablespoon soybean paste (or sub miso paste)
- 2 1/2 tablespoon oyster sauce or vegan oyster sauce

- 1 tablespoon soy sauce

- 2 teaspoons sugar, or honey, maple, coconut sugar

- 2 teaspoons rice wine vinegar

- Water as needed: add in gradually with each step to help prevent protein, eggplants, and vegetables from browning too quickly in the pan.

Instructions

1. Prep Eggplant. Cut the eggplants into long, 1/2-inch thick pieces about 1-2 inches long. Place in a medium bowl, cover with water and 1 teaspoon salt (stir) for 15-20 minutes to keep the eggplants from browning and tasting bitter. Set aside.

2. Make the stir-fry sauce. Mix soybean paste, oyster sauce, soy sauce, sugar, and rice wine vinegar. Set aside for later.

3. Cook the protein: Add a little oil to a large skillet or wok on medium heat. Add a 5-finger pinch of salt. to the oil. Once hot, add chicken or shrimp (see notes for tofu) and cook until lightly browned, and cooked through. Add 2-3 tablespoons of water if necessary to loosen up the pieces in the pan. Once the chicken is cooked,

remove it from the pan and set it aside on a plate. Wipe the skillet lightly with a paper towel.

4. Cook the eggplant: Drain the eggplant, and pat dry with a paper towel. Add 1-2 tablespoons of oil to the pan, then add the eggplant (or spray with spray oil). Cook until the eggplants are caramelized and translucent and tender. Anywhere from 4-7 minutes, depending on the pan you're using. Remove from the pan and set aside with the cooked chicken.

5. Stir fry: Swipe the pan again with a paper towel, then add one tablespoon of oil on medium heat. Add garlic, chilis, and onion, and constantly stir for 2 minutes or until the onion is lightly caramelized. Add 2-3 tablespoons of water if necessary to loosen up the pieces in the pan. You might start to cough from the chilis being fried. It's normal! (A badge of honor when making stir-fries in a Thai kitchen!) (: Turn the vent on or open windows for some air circulation.

6. Add the vegetables (except the basil), stir, and cook for 3-4 more minutes until the vegetables are tender. If using a cast iron pan, they tend to cook everything more quickly because it conducts more heat, so lower heat if necessary. If using a non-stick pan, you may not need to add water at all.

7. Add the cooked chicken and eggplant back into the pan with the vegetables. Stir well and heat through about 2 minutes.

8. Add the stir-fry sauce, and stir for 1-2 more minutes. Taste and adjust the flavors with more soy sauce and a dash of sugar and add more chilis for extra heat.

9. Stir in the fresh basil, saute for 30 seconds, and turn the heat off. The residual heat will continue to cook the basil while not overcooking it. Let it cool for a few minutes. Serve over a plate with rice or carbs of your choice.

11. 30-Minute Thai Green Curry

Prep Time: 15 Minutes

Cook Time: 15 Minutes

Servings: 8

Ingredients

- 1 shallot, finely diced
- 2 tablespoons olive or peanut oil
- 2–4 Tablespoons store-bought green curry paste (see notes) or 1/2 cup homemade green curry paste
- 1 cup veggie or chicken broth
- 1 can coconut milk (full fat)
- 8 ounces extra-firm tofu, cubed (not silken) or chicken breast (thinly sliced- see notes) or shrimp (raw, peeled and de-veined)
- 1/2 teaspoon salt
- 1 teaspoon sugar
- 2 teaspoons fish sauce (or vegan fish sauce)
- 1 Japanese eggplant, thinly sliced into half-moons
- 1 red bell pepper, sliced

- 6–8 kaffir lime leaves
- 1 lime
- 1/4 cup fresh Thai Basil leaves, torn (or sub regular basil)
- Additional lime wedges for garnish
- Other additions or substitutions: snow peas, asparagus, green beans, zucchini, mushrooms, fresh chopped spinach leaves
- Serve over rice or black rice

Instructions

1. Set the rice to cook if using.
2. Heat oil in a heavy bottom pot or dutch oven over medium heat, and saute the shallot. Turn your fan on, and stir-fry green curry paste for 2-3 minutes. Add the broth or stock and scrape up all those delicious browned bits. Add the kaffir lime leaves, and veggies, bring to simmer and cover. (Feel free to add chicken now if using.)
3. Once veggies are just tender (3-5 minutes) stir in the coconut milk, salt, sugar and fish sauce.
4. Add the tofu (or shrimp) and bring to a gentle simmer, simmering uncovered until tofu is warmed through

(and shrimp is cooked- pink and curled) Try to prevent this from coming to a hard boil – a gentle simmer will help preserve the coconut's sweetness.

5. Add a squeeze of lime and taste, adding more lime if needed. If you need more sweetness, add more sugar. More depth, add salt or fish sauce. Find your balance.

6. TIP: Remember you will be serving this over rice, which will mellow out the intensity of flavor- so I like to keep this on the slightly salty/flavorful side.

7. Add the fresh basil leaves and serve with lime wedges over rice.

Prep Time: 20 Minutes

Cook Time: 15 Minutes

Servings: 6

Ingredients

- 1 tablespoon coconut oil
- 1 small red onion, sliced
- 4 garlic cloves, finely chopped
- 2 teaspoons grated ginger
- 2 tablespoons tamarind puree (I used Glory Bee Organic)
- 2 tablespoons fish sauce
- 4 cups vegetable stock or water
- 1 1/2 cups eggplant cut into chunks
- 1 Serrano chili
- 12 ounces fresh salmon filets, cut into large chunks (optional pre-searing if desired)
- 2 heads baby Bok Choy or 2 cups of greens; napa cabbage, spinach, Mizuna
- 1 cup fresh tomatoes (cherry tomatoes are nice), chopped

- 1 tablespoon white miso mixed with 1/4 cup water
- Garnish with fresh cilantro, and thinly sliced daikon radish

Instructions

1. Saute' onion, garlic and ginger in coconut oil for 2 minutes.
2. Add broth, tamarind, fish sauce, eggplant and serrano chili. Bring to a low simmer for 10 minutes, or until eggplant is tender.
3. Add salmon (see notes), tomatoes and Bok Choy (if substituting spinach, wait and add just before serving), cook another 5 minutes or until salmon is just cooked through. Add miso water mixture.
4. Garnish and serve with rice if desired.

Prep Time: 20 Minutes

Cook Time: 20 Minutes

Servings: 4

Ingredients

- Creamy Polenta
- 4 cups water
- 1 teaspoons sea salt
- 1 cup polenta
- 1–2 tablespoons unsalted butter, or olive oil
- Fresh Greek Relish
- 1 cup tomatoes, chopped about 1 medium
- 1 cup cucumber, about 1 small
- 1/2 cup sweet onion, chopped small
- 1 tablespoon fresh oregano, finely chopped
- 1/2 cup fresh basil, torn into bite size pieces
- 1/3 cup pitted kalamata olives, cut in half
- 1/2 cup cooked chickpeas
- 2 teaspoons sherry vinegar
- 3 tablespoons olive oil
- 1/4 teaspoon sea salt

- Optional- 3-6 oz. feta (sheep feta is preferred)
- Grilled Eggplant
- 2 medium eggplants, cut in 3/4 inch rounds
- Olive oil
- Sea salt

Instructions

Make Polenta:

1. Boil water with salt.
2. Slowly add polenta while whisking. Stir until slightly thickening and fully incorporated.
3. Turn heat to low. Cover and simmer for 20 minutes, stirring 2-3 times.
4. Once polenta has softened, stir in butter or olive oil.

Make the Greek relish:

1. Mix all ingredients together in a medium bowl.

Grill Eggplant:

2. Heat the grill to full high heat.
3. Brush eggplant with olive oil.

4. Turn grill to medium heat and place eggplant on the grill. Close lid for 3- 4 minutes. Flip eggplant over and close lid again for another 3-4 minutes.

5. The eggplant will continue to soften once removed from the heat. You can stack them on top of each other, covered with foil, to continue to cook and soften.

Assemble:

1. Divide polenta among 4 bowls, then top with grilled eggplant and the fresh Greek relish.

Prep Time: 30 Minutes

Cook Time: 20 Minutes

Servings: 3

Ingredients

- 1 large or 2 medium/large eggplants – sliced into ½ inch -¾ inch thick slices
- Olive oil, salt and pepper for grilling
- 3–4 tablespoons Gremolata (Zesty Italian Herb Sauce)
- 1 pint cherry or grape tomatoes, halved
- Drizzle olive oil
- OPTIONAL – crumbled goat or feta cheese
- Serve with cauliflower rice, or this Everyday Quinoa with Lemon Shallots and Herbs

Instructions

2. Preheat Grill to medium high (you can also roast these, see notes)
3. Slice eggplant into ½ inch thick slices. (If you are sensitive to bitterness, salt both sides and let sit for 15

minutes, then rinse with water and pat dry.) Brush both sides with olive oil (and salt if not previously) and grill each side for 4-5 minutes, or until good grill marks appear. Remove from grill and stack them in a baking dish or bowl and cover tightly in foil so they continue to cook all the way through and become translucent.

4. Make the Gremolata.

5. Toss the tomatoes with a pinch of salt, fresh herbs (if you like) a little drizzle of olive oil. (You can also just halve them and leave them plain- the Gremolata has plenty of flavor.)

6. Lay the eggplant steaks down on a serving dish. Spoon a little gremolata over each one. Top with the tomatoes.

7. Add crumbled goat or feta if you like. Serve with Cauliflower Rice or Everyday Quinoa on the side.

Prep Time: 25 Minutes

Cook Time: 25 Minutes

Servings: 4

Ingredients

- 1 cup dry Freekeh
- 2 1/2 cups water
- 1 large eggplant, sliced into 1/4 inch slices
- 1/4 cup mint, chopped
- 1/4 cup dill, chopped
- 1/4 cup Italian parsley, chopped
- 3 scallions, sliced
- 1 tablespoon lemon zest
- 4 tablespoons olive oil
- 3–4 tablespoons lemon juice
- 1/2 teaspoon salt, more to taste
- 1/2 teaspoon pepper
- 1 teaspoon sumac (optional)
- 1/2 teaspoon Aleppo chili flakes (optional)

Yogurt Sauce:

- 1 cup plain thick Greek yogurt (or sub vegan yogurt1 tablespoon lemon juice
- 2 tablespoons fresh chopped dill (or mint, or parsley)
- 1–2 garlic cloves finely minced
- ½ teaspoon sumac (optional)
- 1/4 teaspoon salt, or to taste

Instructions

1. Preheat grill to medium high.
2. Place freekeh and water in a medium pot, bring to a boil, cover, then turn heat to low and simmer 15-20 minutes, until water is absorbed and freekeh is tender.
3. Slice the eggplant and brush or spray with olive oil. Season with salt. Grill both sides, 3-4 minutes until grill marks appear, then wrap in foil to allow them to steam and cook through. Cut the eggplant into bite-sized pieces.
4. Place the cooked freekeh, eggplant, chopped herbs, lemon zest, scallions, olive oil, lemon juice, salt, pepper and spices in a bowl. Toss to combine. Taste and adjust salt and lemon. You want it to taste slightly tart. The smoky flavor will come through as it sits.

5. Place the yogurt sauce ingredients in a small bowl and whisk. (if making the vegan version, you may need to add more lemon)

6. To serve, lather the yogurt dressing on platter, and pile the salad over top. Garnish with torn mint leaves.

7. To pack up for lunch, spead a little yogurt sauce on the bottom of the container, spoon salad over top (or keep it separate).

8. Salad will keep 3-4 days in the fridge, with yogurt dressing on the side.

Prep Time: 20 Minutes

Cook Time: 15 Minutes

Servings: 3

Ingredients

- 1 pound Japanese eggplant (2-3 long purple eggplan)
- Oil for brushing or spraying eggplant
- 1/2 cup red onion, very finely sliced (or sub 1 shallot)
- 1/2 cup red bell pepper, cut into strips
- 1 tablespoon jalapeño, finely diced, more or less as preferred
- 1/3 cup cilantro, chopped
- 1/3 cup green onion, sliced
- 1/4 cup fresh mint, leaves torn
- 1/4 cup roasted peanuts, lightly crushed (optional, sub cashews)
- 1–2 tablespoons of fish sauce, start with one, add more to taste
- 1–2 tablespoons fresh lime juice, start with one, add more to taste
- Salt and white or black pepper, to taste

- Serve with boiled eggs (optional, traditional) and jasmine rice.

Instructions

1. Slice the eggplants in half and brush both sides very lightly with oil. If eggplant is thick, then slice. Grill on high heat for 3-4 minutes on each side- or until the desired doneness. Let cool while preparing the salad.
2. Add all the remaining ingredients to a large mixing bowl, including the fish sauce and lime juice. Mix well.
3. Slice the eggplant into long strips, 3-4 inches long. You can peel some of the skin off the eggplants or leave them on. I left mine on.
4. Add the grilled eggplant to the salad bowl, and mix. Taste and adjust with more lime juice, fish sauce, jalapeno, salt, or white pepper for extra flavor.
5. Garnish with boiled eggs and serve with jasmine rice, or enjoy it by itself as a salad or side dish.

Prep Time: 40 Minutes

Cook Time: 20 Minutes

Servings: 7

Ingredients

- 1 large eggplant, sliced into ¼ inch rounds (see notes)
- 1 loaf of bread- rustic bread, French bread, focaccia bread (10 inch in diameter or equivalent)
- 1 jar roasted peppers (or roast your own pepper)
- ½ cup pesto (store-bought or homemade, see below)
- ½ cup olive tapenade (store bought or homemade, see below)
- 8 ounces fresh mozzarella cheese (optional, sub other cheese, or hummus for vegan option)
- Handful arugula
- Other options – turkey breast, cured Italian meats, artichoke hearts, grilled zucchini, grilled Portobello mushrooms
- Basil Pesto (vegan)
- 3 cloves garlic
- 2 ounces fresh basil leaves (about 1 cup packed down)

- ¼ cup plus 2 tablespoons olive oil

- 2 tablespoons fresh lemon juice

- ¼ cup toasted pinenuts (or sub almonds, smoked almonds are nice too)

- ¼ teaspoon salt

Olive tapenade:

- ¼ cup Italian parsley (packed, or sub basil)

- 2 garlic cloves

- ½ cup kalamata olives (or sub green olives)

- 2 tablespoons olive oil

- 1 tablespoon balsamic vinegar

- 1–2 tablespoons capers

- Pinch chili flakes (optional)

Instructions

1. If using eggplant, preheat grill to med-high heat. (Alternative you can roast the eggplant in 400F oven until golden and tender)

2. Slice the eggplant into ¼ inch disks, brush with olive oil and season with salt.

3. While grill is warming up, make the pesto. Place all ingredients in a food processor and pulse repeatedly

until you achieve desired consistency. Scrape out into a bowl.

4. Using the same food processor (no need to rinse) make the olive tapenade. Add the parsley and garlic first and pulse until uniformly chopped. Then add the remaining ingredients EXCEPT the capers, which you will stir in at the end. Pulse repeatedly until nicely chopped but not smooth. Place in a bowl, stir in capers. Add chili flakes if you like.

5. Grill the eggplant, searing both sides nicely 4-5 minutes each side, turning heat down if it's too hot, then place eggplant slices in a foil packet to steam for a few minutes to cook all the way through. It is imperative your eggplant is cooked through.

6. Cut loaf of bread horizontally in half, leaving a good inch on the bottom layer. Spread the bottom with half the pesto. Build the sandwich on a cutting board if possible. Top with eggplant (salt it now, if needed), roasted peppers, fresh mozzarella, olive tapenade (I used about 3/4) and arugula. Spread the top layer of bread with remaining pesto and place it on top. Press down gently. Either serve right away and cut sections with a sharp knife, or refrigerate it, placing on a layer

of paper towels over a plate or platter. Cover with plastic wrap. Enjoy for the next few days.

Prep Time: 10 Minutes

Cook Time: 30 Minutes

Servings: 4

Ingredients

- 1 small eggplant (1 pound)
- Olive oil, salt and pepper
- Kale Slaw (or make the Everyday Kale Slaw and add fresh herbs)
- 6–7 laminate (or Tuscan) kale leaves – 2 cups shredded (packed)
- 1 bunch Italian parsley
- Handful mint leaves
- ¼ cup finely diced onion
- 2 tablespoons olive oil
- 2 tablespoons lemon juice
- ¼ teaspoon salt
- Optional additions- sliced tomato, radishes, cucumber, feta, and yogurt
- Quick tahini sauce (or sub store bought, tahini sauce or baba ganoush)

- 2 tablespoons tahini paste

- 3 tablespoons hot tap water

- 1 tablespoon lemon juice

- ⅛ Tablespoon salt

- 1 minced garlic clove

- 2– 4 wraps or tortillas (feel free to use gluten free) 8-10 inch

Instructions

1. Preheat oven to 425F

2. Slice eggplant into ¼ inch thick disks.

3. Brush each side with olive oil and season with salt and pepper. Place on a parchment lined sheet pan and roast the oven for 25-30 minutes, flipping over after 20 minutes. While they are baking, make the slaw filling and sauce.

4. Thinly slice the kale into thin ribbons, stacking them first then slicing (see photo). Place in a bowl. Finally chop the parsley and mint, thin stems are ok. Add to the bowl along with the onion. Toss with olive oil, lemon juice, salt and pepper. You want this to be quite "juicy", so if needed add a little more oil and lemon juice in equal portions. You can add radishes and/ or

tomatoes here if you want or sprinkle them over top of the wrap.

5. Whisk together the tahini sauce ingredients in a small bowl.

6. Lightly warm or toast the tortilla or wrap. Spread the inside with tahini sauce. Top with warm eggplant and a huge mound of the dressed greens. Top with tomatoes, radishes and feta if you like.

7. This recipe make 2 enormous wraps or 4 smaller ones. Or three medium ones.

8. Notes: For even more flavor, grill the eggplant during the warm months. Both the eggplant and the kale slaw can be made ahead and refrigerated.

Prep Time: 20 Minutes

Cook Time: 50 Minutes

Servings: 2

Ingredients

- 2 large eggplants (1.5 to 1.75 lbs each)
- 2 garlic cloves, finely minced (use a garlic press)
- 4 tablespoons tahini paste
- 1 tablespoon lemon juice
- 1 teaspoon salt
- Optional: 2 tablespoons plain full-fat yogurt
- Garnishes: olive oil, homemade zaatar spice, dukkah, fresh herbs like parsley, olives, toasted pita bread, or fresh veggies (cucumber, tomato, carrot sticks, bell pepper, etc.).

Instructions

Grill Method:

1. Preheat grill to medium-high or oven to 425 F

2. Make a foil packet with wood chips for smoking. Wrap ½ cup of wood chips (mesquite, alder, and apple) in heavy-duty foil and pierce the top, creating an opening in the foil so smoke can escape. Place this on the grill. See photos.

3. With a sharp pairing knife cut 1-2 inch deep slits into the eggplant, all over especially around the bigger bottom area. This will allow them to cook more evenly, and help the smoke penetrate the eggplant.

4. When the foil packet is smoking, place the eggplant directly on the grill, and close the grill. Turn eggplant every 10 minutes or so and let the skin char. Grill until eggplant has collapsed and feels tender on the inside. This will take about 20 minutes.

5. Place the eggplant along with the smoking foil packet in a large bowl or large pan and cover tightly with foil. Let sit until cool enough to handle about 20 minutes.

6. Save ALL the smoky liquid that is under the eggplant in the bowl. Peel the charred skin off the eggplant and using a knife, chop up the tender flesh. Place the eggplant in a strainer and strain the eggplant flesh for 10 minutes. Discard this liquid. (I know this may seem counter-intuitive – but you will be adding some of the "smoky" liquid from the first bowl back in.)

7. Place the drained eggplant in a mixing bowl. You should have 2 cups (or 2 1/4 cups) of eggplant flesh. If you have less, see notes.

8. Add the tahini paste, garlic, lemon, salt and 1-2 tablespoons (or more to taste) of the smoky liquid reserved from the bowl.

9. Mix, taste, and adjust salt, lemon. For a delicious richness, add 2-3 tablespoons plain yogurt (optional). Stir with a fork until relatively smooth. Refrigerate until serving.

Oven Roasting Method:

1. Preheat oven to 450F (425F if electric oven)

2. Slice eggplants in half, lengthwise and roast with flesh side down, on a parchment-lined sheet pan on the middle rack, until very tender, about 45-60 minutes. Test by piercing the skin with a fork, and continue roasting until flesh is very tender and collapsing. Let cool.

3. Scoop out flesh, drain in a strainer for 10 minutes. You should have about 2 cups, if less, see notes.

4. Mash with a fork and add the remaining ingredients. To achieve the smoky flavor, add a 1/4- ½ teaspoon of liquid smoke.

5. Adjust salt and lemon to taste. Stir in optional yogurt.

6. To serve:

7. Place in a shallow serving bowl, make a circular "well" with the back of a spoon and drizzle with olive oil, and your choice of aleppo chili flakes, zaatar spice, dukkah or sumac.

8. Sprinkle with fresh herbs.

9. Serve with warm pita bread and/or veggies.

Prep Time: 20 Minutes

Cook Time: 30 Minutes

Servings: 3

Ingredients

- 1 medium-large eggplant, sliced ⅓ inch thick
- Olive oil for brushing
- 1 red bell pepper
- 2 garlic cloves- finely minced
- 2 tablespoons balsamic vinegar
- 3 tablespoons olive oil
- 2 tablespoons capers
- ½ teaspoon salt
- ¼ cup Basil leaves, packed, and then cut into ribbons.
- Crostini (optional)
- 1 baguette, sliced ½ inch thick
- Olive oil for brushing

Instructions

1. Heat grill to medium-high heat.

2. Slice eggplant into ⅓ inch thick rounds and brush both sides with olive oil.

3. If making crostini, slice baguette into ½ inch thick disks. Brush both sides with olive oil.

4. Once grill is hot, grill eggplant slices, 4-5 minutes on each side, until noticeable grill marks appear, turning heat to medium if necessary, stack eggplant in a bowl and cover tightly with foil so they steam and cook through.

5. Grill the red pepper on all sides over medium high heat until lightly charred and tender. Place with the eggplant under the foil.

6. Grill the baguette slices. (If making this ahead, wait until close to serving time to grill the bread. Alternatively you make bake the bread on a sheet pan in a 375 F oven until crisp and do this the day before.)

7. Uncover the eggplant and let cool, then dice in to small ⅓ inch prices and place in a medium bowl. Dice the bell pepper. Add the finely minced garlic, balsamic vinegar, olive oil, capers, and salt. Taste and add salt if necessary, remembering the bread will dilute the some of the salt.

8. Right before ready to serve, stir in the basil ribbons. To make ribbons, stack the basil leaves uniformly. Roll up from point end to stem end. Thinly slice the roll.

9. Serve the grilled baguette alongside the eggplant caponata or place a tablespoon or two on each piece of bruschetta, garnishing with more basil.

21. Moroccan Pickled Eggplant

Prep Time: 15 Minutes

Cook Time: 15 Minutes

Servings: 1

Ingredients

- 1 ½ tablespoons kosher salt
- 3 tablespoons sugar
- 1 1/2 cups white vinegar (5 percent acidity)
- 2 ½ Cups water
- 2 tablespoons whole coriander seeds
- 5 large garlic cloves, halved
- 1 ½ lbs assorted baby eggplants, with stems (fairytale eggplant or small Japanese)
- Olive oil and cilantro or parsley for serving
- Optional additions- other whole spices, bay leaves, dried or fresh chilies, chili flakes, sliced onion, etc.

Instructions

1. In a medium pot, bring first 6 ingredients to a simmer.

2. Slit each eggplant from blossom end almost to stem end twice, crosswise, so that eggplant splays into four "fingers" attached to the stem end.

3. Place eggplant in simmering liquid and gently simmer 8-10 minutes or until eggplant is tender. (Bigger ones will obviously take longer, mini ones shorter)

4. Using tongs place eggplant in a jar, stems up, and pour the pickling liquid over top. Refrigerate 12 hours.

5. To serve, place eggplant on a platter, drizzle with olive oil and sprinkle with fresh cilantro or Italian parsley.

6. Makes a one-quart jar, and keeps up to 4 weeks in the fridge.

Prep Time: 20 Minutes

Cook Time: 40 Minutes

Servings: 6

Ingredients

- 1 cup French Green, OR Black lentils, OR Beluga Caviar lentils (do not use a split lentil)
- 3 cups water
- 2 cups diced onions
- 5 cloves garlic, minced
- 1 tablespoon fresh ginger, minced
- 1 cup diced carrot
- 1 cup diced tomato
- 2–3 tablespoons Berbere Spice Mix
- 1 teaspoon salt
- 2 tablespoon olive oil
- Fresh Italian parsley for garnish

Berbere Chicken:

- 6 chicken thighs (skin-on)
- 2–3 tablespoons Berbere Spice Mix

- Olive oil

- Kosher Salt

- Berbere Spice Mix

- 3 tablespoons paprika

- 1 tablespoon red pepper flakes, ground plus more for extra spicy

- 2 teaspoons cumin seeds or powdered cumin

- 1 teaspoon coriander seeds or powdered coriander

- 1 teaspoon cardamom seeds (shelled) or powdered cardamom

- 1 teaspoon turmeric

- 1 teaspoon salt

- 1 teaspoon fenugreek seeds or powdered fenugreek

- 1 teaspoon black peppercorns or freshly ground peppercorn

- 1/2 teaspoon ground cloves

- 1/2 teaspoon allspice

- 1/2 teaspoon ground ginger

- 1/2 teaspoon cinnamon

Instructions

1. Preheat oven to 400 F

2. Make the lentils: In a heavy bottom pot, or dutch oven, saute diced onion, carrots, garlic and ginger in 2 tablespoons olive oil, until tender, about 5-7 minutes. Add 2-3 tablespoons Berbere Spice mix and sauté 2-3 minutes. Add 1 cup lentils, 1 cup diced tomatoes, 1 teaspoon salt and 3 cups water, and bring to a boil, cover, turn heat to low and let cook until tender, about 30 minutes. Uncover and cook off any extra liquid.

3. Make the Chicken: Pat dry the chicken and salt all sides with salt and pepper and generously rub each piece with Berbere Spice Mix. The more, the spicier.

4. Heat 1 tablespoon oil in a heavy bottom skillet, on medium-high heat, place chicken skin side down and sear until it is crispy and golden, about 6- 8 minutes. Turn over, and turn heat down to medium, searing for 2-3 minutes. Place in a 400 F oven until internal temperature reaches 165F (10-15 minutes)

5. Serve over a bed of the Ethiopian lentils, and garnish with fresh Italian parsley.

Berbere Spice Mix:

1. If using whole seeds, lightly toast them on the stovetop in a skillet for 2-3 minutes.

2. Grind them using a coffee grinder or mortar and pestle. Remember to crush or grind the chili flakes.

Prep Time: 10 Minutes

Cook Time: 30 Minutes

Servings: 4

Ingredients

- 3 tablespoons ghee (or coconut oil, but ghee will elevate)
- 1 large onion, diced
- 4 cloves garlic, rough chopped
- 2 tablespoons ginger, finely chopped
- 1 medium jalapeno, finely chopped (or 1 Serrano) this is mildly spicy, add more if you like.
- 1/2 teaspoon fennel seeds
- 1 teaspoon black mustard seeds
- 2 teaspoon cumin seeds
- 2 teaspoons garam masala
- 1 lb BABY spinach (fresh or frozen)
- 20 fresh mint leaves
- 1 teaspoon dried fenugreek leaves
- 2 tablespoons water (if using fresh spinach)
- 3/4 cup water

- 1/2 cup plain yogurt (or vegan yogurt)

- 3 –4 cups cooked black lentils (or aka caviar lentils, beluga lentils or French green lentils)

- 1 teaspoon salt, more to taste!

Instructions

1. If cooking black lentils and basmati rice, start them first (see notes)

2. Make the Spinach Sauce: Sautee the onion in ghee, in a large pan, over medium heat for 3-4 minutes, then add garlic, ginger and chilies. Saute until fragrant and golden. Add the fennel seeds, mustard seeds, cumin seeds and garam masala and stir two minutes. Lower heat to low. Add the fresh spinach, fresh mint, fenugreek and 2 tablespoons water. Cover pan, 2-3 minutes, letting spinach wilt. Give a few stirs. Don't overcook!

3. Blend Spinach Sauce: Place the wilted spinach mixture in a blender and add the 3/4 cups of water. Pulse and few times (hold the lid down tight). If you want a smooth sauce, blend until smooth. I left a little texture here. Pour it back into the pan, set on low heat. Don't overheat or you will lose the pretty color.

4. Combine: Stir in the yogurt, lentils and salt. Taste. Adjust salt to your liking, adding more if necessary! You want this slightly more salty because you are serving over rice which will mellow it out a lot. For more heat add a pinch of cayenne or chili flakes. To "up" the flavor even more, add a bit more garam masala spice to taste. If you want a little acidity a tiny squeeze of lemon is nice.

5. Serve with the basmati rice and naan bread!

6. Emerald Dal will keep up to 4 days in the fridge.

Prep Time: 30 Minutes

Cook Time: 45 Minutes

Servings: 8

Ingredients

- 2 1/2 lbs potatoes (Yukon gold, red, or any thin-skinned) (OR use 5 cups leftover mashed potatoes, with curry powder)
- 4 tablespoons, ghee, butter, vegan butter (ghee tastes the BEST)
- 1/2 cup plain yogurt (or sour cream)
- 1/2 cup milk (or nut milk), half and half or heavy cream
- 1 teaspoon salt, more to taste
- 1/2 teaspoon pepper
- 1–2 teaspoons yellow curry powder, more to taste
- Filling
- 2 1/2 cups cooked lentils (3/4 cup -1 cup dry)
- 2 tablespoons ghee, or olive oil
- 1 large onion, diced
- 4 cloves garlic, rough chopped
- 2 cups diced carrot, (2–3 carrots)

- 2 cups diced celery (2–3 ribs)
- 2 teaspoons garam masala, more to taste
- 1 teaspoon cumin
- 1 teaspoon coriander
- 1 teaspoon salt
- 1/2 teaspoon pepper
- 2 teaspoons dried fenugreek leaves
- 1 cup veggie broth
- 1 cup frozen peas (or corn, or green beans- or use fresh)

Gravy:

- 2 tablespoon ghee or olive oil
- 1 teaspoon cumin seeds
- 1 teaspoon fennel seeds
- 3 tablespoons flour (or gf flour)
- 1 1/4 cups warm veggie broth
- Optional garnish: scallions, chives, or cilantro

Instructions

1. Preheat oven to 350F
2. Cook Potatoes: Cut potatoes in one-inch slices (if small, just in half) and place in a large pot. Cover with one-

inch salted water. Bring to a boil, lower heat, cover and simmer until very tender about 20-25 minutes.

3. Cook lentils: Set lentils to cook in salted water (unless cooked already – and you could absolutely do this ahead) about 20-25 minutes (see notes) simmer until tender, but not falling apart, al dente.

4. Make the filling: In a large 10-12 inch ovenproof skillet (or wide, shallow dutch oven) -heat the ghee over medium high heat and saute the onion 2-3 minutes, lower heat to med, add garlic, saute 2 minutes, add carrots, celery, cook 5-7 minutes. Add salt, cumin, coriander, fenugreek leaves and garam masala.

5. Add broth. Bring to a simmer, cover and simmer on med low, until carrots are cooked through about 7-8 minutes.

6. While this is simmering, MAKE THE GRAVY: Over medium heat, in a little pot, simmer the whole seeds (cumin seeds and fennel seeds) in ghee or oil until fragrant and golden. Add flour, whisking, stirring and toasting the flour one minute. Gradually whisk in the warm veggie broth. Cook until slightly thickened. Add this gravy to the filling, along with the peas and drained lentils. Mix to combine.

7. Taste the filling and adjust salt and pepper. Add more garam masala if you like. The filling should have thick stew-like, saucy consistency. If too dry, add a splash of broth or water. If too watery, simmer off some of that liquid. If the filling is too watery, the mashed potatoes will sink.

8. Mash the potatoes: Drain the potatoes (saving some hot potato water) return to the same pot and mash with the 3-4 tablespoons ghee and yogurt. If potatoes seem dry or too stiff, add a little warm potato water to loosen. If you want extra richness a little milk, nut milk, half and half, or whipping cream is nice. I add about ½ cup. (Adding more yogurt will make these too tangy.) Season with salt, pepper and curry powder. Mash and whip until relatively smooth and light and fluffy. Taste and adjust salt.

9. ASSEMBLE: Place 8 big dollops over the lentils stew and fill in the spaces with smaller spoonfuls, carefully spreading out, maybe making a pattern with the back of the spoon, like frosting a cake.

10. Place in the oven until golden and bubbling, about 20-25 minutes. Feel free to brown the top under a broiler.

11. Garnish with scallions, chives or cilantro.

Prep Time: 20 Minutes

Cook Time: 45 Minutes

Servings: 6

Ingredients

- 3 tablespoons olive oil, butter or ghee
- 1 cup diced red onion (1/2 a red onion)
- 1 cup diced carrot
- 1/2 cup diced celery
- 1 cup peeled and diced beet (one large beet, plus 2 more for juicing-optional)
- 4 cloves garlic-rough chopped
- 1 tablespoon fresh thyme leaves
- 1 Bay leaf
- 1 1/2 cups black caviar lentils, beluga lentils or Puy lentils (soaked overnight if possible)
- 4 cups vegetable stock (or chicken stock)
- 1/2 teaspoon salt, more to taste
- 1 tablespoon balsamic vinegar, more to taste
- 1 cup fresh beet juice (either purchase from a juice bar, or juice 2 extra-large beets) or sub more broth or stock

- Optional Garnishes 2- 3 tablespoons browned butter (optional but delicious) or crumbled goat cheese

Instructions

1. In a large heavy bottom pot or dutch oven, heat olive oil over medium high heat. Add onion, carrot, beets and celery, and saute for 5 minutes, until slightly softened.

2. Turn heat to medium, add garlic and herbs and sauté for 2 more minutes. Add lentils, stock and salt and bring to a boil. Once boiling, cover with lid, and turn heat to low, maintaining a gentle simmer. Simmer for 25 minutes or until lentils are just tender.

3. Add the beet juice, taste for salt, add more if necessary, and continue simmering on low for 10-15 more minutes or until tender. If you feel there is too much liquid for your liking, keep the lid off, and increase the heat, letting it reduce. (I like this braise slightly juicy, personally, so I just replace the lid.)

4. Stir in the balsamic vinegar and taste again, adjusting if necessary.

5. Serve with optional browned butter or goat cheese crumbles. If going vegan, a little drizzle of olive oil is nice.

6. Serve as vegan main dish or as a side dish to fish, chicken or meat.

Prep Time: 15 Minutes

Cook Time: 30 Minutes

Servings: 2

Ingredients

- 8–10 ounces Ahi tuna (2 x 4–5 ounce pieces or equivalent)
- 1 Tablespoon fennel seeds
- 1 Tablespoon cumin seeds
- 1 teaspoon granulated garlic
- ¼ teaspoon chili flakes
- ¼ teaspoon salt
- ½ teaspoon cracked pepper
- 2–3 tablespoons oil (olive, coconut)
- Seasoned Lentils
- 1 cup black lentils – beluga or black caviar
- 2 3/4 cups water
- ¾ teaspoon salt
- 1 teaspoon granulated garlic
- 1 teaspoon coriander
- 1 tablespoon olive oil

- Squeeze of lemon

- Moroccan Roasted Carrots

- 2 tablespoons chopped Italian parsley, dill or cilantro

- Drizzle plain yogurt- optional

Instructions

1. Set lentils to boil with water, salt and spices in a medium pot. Once boiling, cover and simmer on low heat until cooked through about 20-25 minutes. Uncover and let any extra liquid reduce for a few minutes. Drizzle with olive oil. Adjust salt and add a squeeze of lemon.

2. Mix ahi spices together in a wide shallow bowl. Cut ahi no thinner than one inch thick at thinnest point. Heat a generous amount of oil in a cast iron skillet, over medium high heat.

3. Coat all sides of the ahi in the spice mix.

4. When pan is smoking (you want the oil to be very hot), very carefully, slowing lay the Ahi in the hot oil. Using a splatter guard, protect yourself from popping seeds. You can also use a lid, but make sure to leave it partially open (you don't want ahi to steam or over cook)

5. Sear each side about 1 -2 minutes or until golden. You want the edges seared just until golden and crispy, but the middle cooked rare. Set aside and slice.

6. Plate the lentils, drizzle with plain yogurt and top with the Moroccan Roasted Carrots and Ahi.

7. Sprinkle with fresh herbs.

Prep Time: 20 Minutes

Cook Time: 20 Minutes

Servings: 11

Ingredients

- 1 onion, diced (or sub 2 fat shallots)
- 8 cloves garlic, rough chopped
- 3 tablespoons olive oil
- 4 cups diced veggies – any mix of carrots, celery, fennel, parsnip, bell pepper, and potato, cabbage (I normally use 2 carrots, 2 celery, 1 parsnip or bell pepper)
- 1 1/2– 2 teaspoons salt, more to taste.
- 1 tablespoon cumin
- 2 teaspoons coriander
- 2 teaspoons curry powder
- 1 teaspoon turmeric
- 1/2 teaspoon allspice (optional)
- 1 bay leaf or 1 teaspoon herbs de Provence or Italian herbs
- 1 tablespoons tomato paste

- 2 medium tomatoes, diced with their juices (or 14 - ounce can of diced tomatoes with juices)
- 4 flavorful cups veggie stock (or chicken stock- use 3 bouillon cubes w/ water)
- 2 cups water
- 1 ¼ cup small Black Caviar lentils or French Green Lentils (You can always use bigger, brown lentils, but increase pressure cooking time to 20 minutes.) You can also substitute split lentils for ¼ cup of the lentils for a creamier texture.
- Garnishes: with a drizzle of olive oil, lemon juice, chopped Italian parsley (or cilantro), diced tomatoes and optional chili flakes (Aleppo chili is nice here) and
- Serve with warm toasty pita bread.

Instructions

1. See notes for stovetop.
2. Saute onion and garlic in the Instant Pot in 2 tablespoons oil until fragrant and tender, about 2-3 minutes.
3. Add the veggies. Saute 4-5 more minutes. Add the spices, salt and tomato paste and brown it a bit. Add

the tomatoes and their juices, stock and water, scraping up any browned bits.

4. Add the lentils, stir and cover, setting the Instant pot to Pressure Cook on Normal for 12 minutes.

5. Let the pressure release either manually or naturally.

6. Taste, adjust salt, adding more to taste.

7. Divide among bowls and drizzle with olive oil, a squeeze of lemon, chili flakes, fresh parsley and fresh diced tomato (optional)

Prep Time: 15 Minutes

Cook Time: 20 Minutes

Servings: 6

Ingredients

- 3 tablespoons ghee or coconut oil
- 1/2 teaspoon whole cumin seeds
- 1/2 teaspoon whole coriander seeds
- 1/2 teaspoon whole mustard seeds
- 1 onion, chopped
- 3 garlic cloves, roughly chopped
- 1 teaspoon grated ginger
- 1 Serrano chili, slit in half leaving the stem intact
- 1 tablespoon yellow curry powder
- 1 carrot, chopped
- 1 yam, cubed
- 1 green apple, cubed
- 4 cups vegetable or chicken broth
- 1/2 cup red lentils
- 1 teaspoon sea salt
- 1 tomato, chopped

- 15 ounces coconut milk
- 1/4 cup fresh parsley, chopped
- 1/4 cup fresh cilantro- leaves and stems, chopped
- 1–3 teaspoons fresh lemon juice

Instructions

1. Turn instant pot on saute function. Add ghee and cumin, mustard, coriander seeds. Saute 2 minutes.
2. Add onion, garlic, ginger, the slit Serrano chili, and curry powder. Saute 3 more minutes.
3. Add carrot, yam, apple, broth, red lentils, sea salt, tomato, and coconut milk. Stir and scrape any bits stuck on the bottom. Set the instant pot to medium pressure for 10 minutes.
4. Release the pressure. Stir in parsley, cilantro and lemon juice.
5. Serve with yogurt and naan bread or basmati rice.

Prep Time: 15 Minutes

Cook Time: 15 Minutes

Servings: 8

Ingredients

- 2 tablespoons olive oil
- One onion, diced
- 5–6 garlic cloves, rough chopped
- 3 carrots, diced (2 cups) (or sub other root veggies- yam or sweet potato, parsnips, celery root, sun chokes)
- 1 red bell pepper, diced
- 1 poblano pepper, diced (optional, for a subtle heat)
- One 14-ounce can diced tomatoes (or sub 1 1/2 cups diced tomatoes with juices)
- 4 cups veggie broth (or chicken broth)
- 1 1/2 teaspoon salt
- 2 teaspoons cumin
- 1 teaspoon chili powder
- 1 teaspoon coriander
- 1 teaspoon cinnamon
- 1 teaspoon dried thyme (or add a few bay leaves)

- 1/2 teaspoon turmeric

- 1 teaspoon maple syrup (or honey)

- 3/4 cup red lentils (split lentils)

- 1/4 cup quinoa

- Optional additions: 1/4 cup raisins

- Garnish: fresh cilantro, parsley, scallions or mint, a squeeze of lemon or lime, a drizzle of olive oil (or swirl of yogurt) or even sliced avocado.

Instructions

1. See notes for the stovetop.

2. Set Instant Pot (Pressure cooker) to saute function and heat the oil. Add the onion and garlic and saute 3-4 minutes, stirring until fragrant. Add the carrots, bell pepper and optional poblano and stir 2 minutes.

3. Add the diced tomatoes (and juices) and broth. Stir in the salt, cumin, chili powder, coriander, cinnamon, turmeric, thyme, and maple syrup. Stir in the split red lentils and the quinoa. You will be tempted to add more but don't. Give a good stir. At this point, you could also toss in 1/4 cup raisins (or add after).

4. Set instant pot to high pressure for 5 minutes.
    Manually release (cover the spout with a kitchen
    towel).

5. Taste, adjust salt if needed. For a bit of acid, a squeeze
    of lemon or lime is nice. The stew will thicken as it sits.

6. Serve this up with fresh radishes and herbs. Add a
    drizzle of olive oil (or for extra richness and a swirl of
    yogurt).

Prep Time: 10 Minutes

Cook Time: 30 Minutes

Servings: 4

Ingredients

- 2 teaspoons olive oil
- 1 shallot, finely chopped
- 3–4 garlic cloves, rough chopped
- ½ cup dry whole lentils (the smallest lentils cook the fastest- I like Black Caviar, and do not use split lentils)
- 4 cups veggie stock
- 1 teaspoon salt, more to taste
- 1 teaspoons cumin
- 1 teaspoon coriander
- 2–3 cups grated raw beets (2 tennis ball-sized beets, peeled, grated). FYI You can sometimes find grated beets in the "salad bar" section of upscale grocery stores.
- 1 lemon
- Garnish- fresh herbs (dill, flat-leaf parsley or cilantro) drizzle of olive oil, pomegranate seeds (optional).

Instructions

1. Heat oil in medium pot over medium heat. Sauté shallot for 2-3 minutes, then add garlic. Saute 2 more minutes until golden and fragrant. Add stock, lentils, beets (save a little for fresh garnish) salt and cumin and coriander. Bring to a simmer, then cover and cook on low simmer, for 30 minutes or until lentils are cooked through and tender. If using larger lentils you will need to cook longer, so keep simmering, covered until tender.
2. When lentils are tender, squeeze in the juice from one lemon.
3. Taste and adjust salt and spices to your liking.
4. Divide among 2 bowls. Top with a handful of fresh grated beets and fresh dill (or cilantro, parsley) and drizzle with a little olive oil. Add a few fresh pomegranate seeds if you like.